YOGA SECRETS REVEALED

The Ultimate Guide to Loving Yoga

Rebecca K. Nelson

Table Of Contents

Introduction

Yoga is something different to most people. It's pretty diverse, and practitioners have different expectations when they start. That's perfectly okay. Whether your goal is greater enlightenment, a more toned and muscular body, or relief from disease, there's Yoga for you. This b00k will serve as a guide.

The philosophy of Yoga has been around for 5,000 years. That's an undeniable staying power. Yoga is not just an 'exercise'; it is a philosophy, a way of thinking rather than a religion. In ancient India, the word yoga meant union. It refers to a collaboration of the entire self – mind, body, and spirit.

This union is achieved through physical poses, frequently called asanas, although asana is just one of the many types of Yoga. These poses are meant to heighten mind and body awareness, making Yoga a natural corollary to meditation.

Today's researchers are discovering the many benefits of Yoga. While it can increase spirituality, it also can heal many ailments and diseases, especially stress, immune system disorders, and heart problems. It also provides increased flexibility, which can reverse the aging process.

The more vigorous yoga practices are considered cardiovascular exercises. Along with a proper diet, you will be able to lose weight. The gentler types of Yoga do not have cardiovascular benefits, so remember to do additional exercises.

Why are people becoming interested in Yoga? The most common reason is to improve flexibility and physical health. Besides the physical benefits, Yoga also boosts mental power and paves the way to spiritual enlightenment. For most, it's the spiritual awakening that turns Yoga into an essential part of their lives. This is a gradual but excellent development and opportunity for personal growth. The essence of Yoga is always to become a better version of oneself.

Chapter 1:

What is the Science

Of Yoga?

People have been practicing Yoga for thousands of years. While the original purpose was to elevate to a greater spiritual level, it became clear that Yoga benefits the person as a whole. Modern scientific research has shown that the tremendous overall health benefits of a yoga lifestyle.

Yes, Yoga does improve the body, but surprising scientific research has shown that it changes the brain. It's about becoming a better version of yourself and getting in touch with the real, authentic you as the brain becomes more uncluttered. It keeps us focused on the present. While Yoga begins on the mat, it extends to our entire day as greater compassion and awareness become a part of our lives.

Yoga won't provide untold riches, although the physical benefits are remarkable. The world is already filled with abundance, much of which we ignore. The natural beauty of Yoga is that it grounds us to the present, connecting us to the mess that is within our grasp. A better, more fulfilled life is within our reach when we let go and accept what is there.

Each yoga pose, which usually involves stretches, has its purpose and benefit. The practitioner becomes aware of the tension and learns to release it. Yoga poses are particular, and perfection comes with practice, but it is not the ultimate goal. Yoga involves a lot of stretching, but, more importantly, it creates balance by increasing flexibility and strength. Whatever type of Yoga you practice, your body and mind simply improve.

Yoga is highly diverse and individual, making it essential to work at your level of comfort. Don't use the person next to you in class as a guide or even the teacher. Work the poses in the best way for you. This isn't a speed contest, and you have nothing to prove. Yoga is a lifetime commitment, not a competition.

Even if you are not used to exercising, you can practice Yoga. You may not be as flexible as the next person, but you will get there. Yoga is always a work in progress and never a competition. While it is a physical practice, Yoga will inevitably touch on your spiritual side. It unifies mind and body to become one.

Research conducted throughout the 20th century has found a myriad of physical benefits to practicing Yoga.

Relief from Stress

Our lives are filled with daily stressors, and we know that stress can cause tremendous damage to the body and mind. The boss wants to talk, your spouse is upset, the mortgage is overdue, and the kids enjoy the keys to the car. Just another typical day.

Holding yoga poses, stretching muscles, being focused on the presents, and breathing deeply and slowly helps us achieve a state of greater relaxation and harmony. We can consciously choose our response to stress instead of being at its mercy. Remaining calm under challenging circumstances is a choice, and Yoga can provide the tools.

Yoga and Pain Relief

Studies have proven that practicing Yoga can provide tremendous relief for people who have multiple sclerosis, arthritis, and other chronic conditions. We'll discuss its fantastic effect on the auto-immune system and cardio system at greater length in other chapters.

Yoga and Breathing

Yoga combines physical movements with breathing. Slower, deeper breathing can alleviate stress.

Yoga and Flexibility

Yoga involves a lot of stretching, which strengthens muscles. Since Yoga impacts the entire body, flexibility, and elasticity from head to toe, it also loosens tight, tense muscles and helps us become more relaxed.

Yoga and Weight Management

Yoga does not burn up as many calories as some other exercise regimes. However, it does increase body awareness. People who practice Yoga become more aware of what they eat and its effect upon their health.

This usually leads to better, healthier eating habits and a natural loss of unwanted weight.

Yoga and Circulation

If your blood isn't supplying your body and brain properly with oxygen, your health will suffer. You need proper circulation for the brain to function, energy, and the growth of cells. Sluggish circulation can cause nerve and tissue damage, blood clots, dizziness, among other problems.

The thorough stretching in most yoga poses will improve circulation. The Camel Pose described in this book is an excellent way to improve circulation.

Yoga and Cardio Health

For patients who have experienced heart surgery, depression and anxiety can be a natural result. Yoga can help manage this type of post-operative stress. It can also lower blood pressure, serving as a heart-healthy preventive measure. The specific heart benefits will be discussed in a separate chapter.

There's No Hurry – Take Your Time

These benefits will take time to achieve. Yoga is not a two-week miracle program. So, as you begin with your yoga sessions, allow sufficient time for the results to manifest themselves. You should see a massive difference in approximately two months. Whatever your reason for practicing Yoga, you should notice an improvement in all aspects of your being.

Chapter 2:
The Ancient History
of Yoga

Yoga has become quite trendy these days as practitioners in their yoga pants and mat head toward the famous yoga studios to attend their weekly yoga sessions. Many of these fashionable yogis are probably unaware of the long history of Yoga dating back to ancient times in India and its spiritual roots.

Most of what we think of as Yoga only dates back 150 years. While people today practice yoga for their health, its roots are entwined in rich spiritualism that took a lifetime to master. For ancient yogis, Yoga was a way of life.

Mention of Yoga first appeared around 1500 BC in Hindu literature. In the first writings, in traditional Sanskrit, the term yoga, which means yoke, frequently refers to a dying warrior rising to heaven and reaching a higher power. The original concept of Yoga was clearly to elevate those who deserved it to a higher level, to connect the individual to the universe as a whole.

For ancient Buddhists, Yoga wasn't even a specific discipline. It grew out of the desire to attain spiritual goals and control both the mind and the body to achieve this.

These spiritual leaders recognized that man is fallible but always capable of improvement by changing dysfunctional thinking. They recognized the power of the mind to bring about inner peace and alleviate suffering by broadening individual consciousness and becoming open to new ideas. They already understood the basics of the mind/body connection.

Yoga, including meditation, was and still is a quest for knowledge. Ancient practitioners thought, correctly, as it turns out, that knowledge would lead to a higher level of consciousness and existence.

Old writings describe several levels of being, increasing knowledge bringing the practitioner to the next, higher level. It was viewed as a process that, for many, encompassed a lifetime of learning. Yoga, the physical part of gaining enlightenment, was to prepare meditation, which was spiritual. The physical side of Yoga began to emerge around 500 AD.

By the third century, Yoga was an accepted Buddhist practice involving a spiritual quest through meditation. This is the classical period, where the writings Vyasa introduced the all-important Yoga Sutras, which lists Yoga as a precondition for a higher existence. For several centuries, the practice of Yoga became an accepted practice to attain critical personal values, although it was still far from today's set of poses.

More meditative, it was intended to help "transcend" human suffering and rise above it. It was also used to broaden or deepen consciousness as a path to personal enlightenment. Yoga was seen as a means to overcome destiny and regain control of the self. The beginning of training and controlling the mind is emerging.

Up to the 15th century, while the West was in constant strife and war, Eastern Buddhism focused on peace of mind. The difference between a Western and Eastern mindset is becoming more noticeable. By this time, the emphasis on yoga shifts from transcending pain to reaching a higher plane of existence. Man himself is to become a deity.

By the eighth century, Hatha Yoga, a mix of poses and meditation, came into practice. It is the beginning of "modern" Yoga as we know it today.

Modern Yoga

Yoga, the old spiritual quest of Buddhism, didn't reach the West until the last 19th century. This coincided with an interest in

Indian culture as a whole due to the burgeoning spice trade.

Western culture became intrigued by the writings of Swami Vivekananda, a monk. He traveled to Europe and introduced the intelligentsia to Buddhist spiritual writings, especially the 4th century Yoga Sutras, which involve clearing the mind of unwanted thoughts and learning to focus on one thing.

As we know it today, Yoga became popular in the U.S. in the 1940s, when young Americans began to take yoga classes. By the 1980s, the known health benefits of Yoga increased its popularity, although the practice was seen as more physical than spiritual by the majority of practitioners.

By the 21st century, the devotees of American Yoga have increased from 4 million at the turn of the century to 20 million by 2011. This increase in popularity is mainly due to the increased scientific studies of the numerous benefits of Yoga, especially the alleviation of stress. Whether spiritual or not, people want to increase their health. Many people, however, still seek both mental *and* physical elevation. Yoga offers both.

While mastering the physical aspects of Yoga is essential, it is equally crucial not to lose sight of the spiritual benefits. Yoga is more than posting adorable selfies on Instagram.

Thousands of years ago, Yoga was a preparation for the spiritual enlightenment of meditation. It was intended to prepare and relax the body for meditative practice. It is important not to lose sight of that.

To achieve your spiritual side, keep in mind the Seven Spiritual Laws of Yoga:

1. You have unlimited potential. The purpose of Yoga is to reach a high level of consciousness.

2. The universe is filled with abundance. To receive, learn to give.

3. Understand the universal law of cause and effect, known as karma. Your actions, whether positive or negative, will be returned in equal measure.

4. Don't resist life's forces. Your desires will manifest themselves when you most minor fight.

5. Be clear on what your desires and intentions are.

6. Stop struggling and remain open to all opportunities that come your way.

7. Know what your true purpose in life is.

Meditation, which will be discussed in the final chapter of this book, will help you achieve the spiritual laws of Yoga.

Chapter 3:

Establishing the

Mind/Body Connection

with Yoga

The purpose of Yoga has always been to connect the mind to the body. That is what the Buddhists had in mind thousands of years ago. Even then, it was clear that when the mind and body work as one, the self becomes healthier, more aware, and can function at a higher level.

But how exactly is the mind and body connected? People who are aware of their thoughts and feelings can cope with stress and life's adversities better. They form better and healthier relationships.

Ultimately, they believe in their ability to succeed.

We all face setbacks. It's how we handle them that makes the difference.

Emotional wellbeing is rarely a constant, however. Unexpected events can lead to depression, anxiety, stress, and confusion.

Losing a job, physical injury, the death or injury of someone we love, or the end of a relationship can cause emotional upheaval. Even good events, such as a new home, marriage, or a new job, can cause anxiety as we face the unknown.

When our mind experiences turmoil, the body immediately responds. If you needed a reminder, the body is there to tell you that all is not well. The body does that in some ways, such as developing high blood pressure, ulcers, insomnia, etc. These symptoms are all physical manifestations of an anxious mind. Whether we realize it or not, the mind and body work as a team.

So, where does Yoga come into play?

As Yoga increases our mental awareness, we become more aware of underlying emotions and thoughts. That allows us to express and acknowledge them rather than keeping them buried and allowing them to fester. Appropriately expressing negative emotions will enable us to deal with them and put them behind us.

When we deal effectively with negativity, we can acknowledge the more positive aspects of our lives. Sometimes, we can become so overwhelmed, we no longer see anything good or positive, even if it is all around us. Yoga provides that necessary balance. Yes, work can be stressful, but we see more to our lives than that. This is a healthy outlook that boosts the overall quality of our life when we need it.

A healthy mind/body connection allows us to cope with adversity as we become more resilient. Resilience is a skill that can be learned and developed. It prevents us from being victims of circumstances and gives us greater control over our lives. We can strengthen our resilience through relaxation and creating a calmer outlook.

Both Yoga and meditation are invaluable tools for taking greater control over our thoughts, feelings, and our life in general. When we are in control, we sleep better, eat healthier, and connect with others on a higher level.

Our emotional health invariably affects our immune system, as we will see in another chapter. A weakened immune system can leave the body vulnerable to colds, inflammations, and infections.

The myriad ways that the mind impacts the body became more apparent during the 20th century when repeated studies reveal how stress and emotions can become inevitably linked and connected. Thankfully, modern physicians are taking a more integrated approach to their patients' health. More are recommending Yoga and meditation not only for stress but for cardiovascular diseases, all well.

Discuss the overall benefits of Yoga with your doctor whenever the state of your mental and physical health can continually be enhanced.

Chapter 4:

Yoga – Strength and Flexibility

Strength training, usually in the form of lifting weights or Cross Fit, has been gaining popularity. Women especially are appreciating a more toned, muscled, and muscular body.

Increasing bodily strength is essential to prevent osteoporosis and the natural loss of muscles as we age. Strong muscles help keep joints healthy and prevent injuries.

While the benefits of strength training are clear, some people question whether practicing Yoga counts toward increasing strength and muscles. This may be especially the case for athletic males, who

32

view Yoga as a "girlie" activity. But can Yoga build strength and muscles?

It depends on the type of Yoga you practice. Certain types of Yoga are deliberately gentle. Restorative Yoga falls into that category. This doesn't make them any less effective; it merely means more people, especially older ones, can enjoy Yoga's benefits. As we've discussed, Yoga is for everyone.

However, yoga exercises are demanding and challenging and would be difficult for even a strong male. Poses such as Planks and Warrior require the support of the entire body and will undoubtedly develop muscles and strength. These poses strengthen the whole body, not just specific muscles that would get a workout during weightlifting. The poses can be done with small hand weights for maximum results. Thus, Yoga can be better at building strength than some other forms of exercise.

Ashtanga and Vinyasas Yoga can increase strength through more significant poses, especially in the upper body and legs. In addition, holding poses for a more extended period, such as up to two minutes per pose, is a fantastic muscle enhancer. Just keep in mind it takes time to build that type of stamina.

But building muscles is an individual goal. How much muscle is enough? For maximum muscle-building, weights can certainly help bring about quicker results. Many people use both Yoga and weightlifting for some dramatic bulking up.

Unlike weight training, Yoga isn't specifically geared toward the physique. It is much more than exercise.

With weightlifting, you can build muscles indefinitely by simply adding additional weights. If you wish, you can build isolated muscles such as your thighs into the size of a tree trunk. With Yoga, you build strength more balanced way as all muscles, big and small, are built up. The emphasis is on power rather than bulk. Your body becomes more resilient and allows you to use that strength in all physical activities, such as lifting, twisting, and bending. Instead of a more muscular person, you become a stronger individual.

You can incorporate other exercises into your yoga program. But Yoga itself, when practiced regularly, will continue to improve your body and add strength and flexibility.

Yoga stretches are widely known for improving flexibility. Flexibility and balance become especially important as we age and become vulnerable to injuries. Many people believe that you need to be flexible *before* starting a yoga practice, but the opposite is true. You can begin Yoga in any physical condition and keep improving your flexibility.

Three specific areas of the body are frequently tight: the hips, shoulders, and hamstrings. We spend a lot of our time inactive and sitting, and these muscles can become relatively inflexible through non-use.

Daily yoga stretches will increase your flexibility tremendously as you provide these muscle groups with a real workout. As always, don't stretch your muscles to the point of pain. Stretch to the limit of your comfort, and you will soon see the results.

Now, let's discuss another muscle that can be inflexible, namely the brain. Yes, the brain is indeed a muscle. If you have rigid attitudes, such as that things should be done only one way, you limit your mental power. Perhaps your mind is frequently made up about specific issues, and you see no reason to explore them further. The purpose of Yoga is to unleash your mental powers. It involves a change in *all* areas of your life. Yoga is a vast four-letter word.

The combination of Yoga and meditation opens up the mind to new ideas and ways of doing things. It encourages curiosity. Many people hold on to old, traditional beliefs because of fear. Yoga is meant to alleviate that fear and open up new, life-enhancing possibilities.

When it comes to Yoga, you will soon enjoy a more flexible body, as well as a mind that becomes open, flexible, and curious.

Chapter 5:

Managing Weight

with Yoga

It is a well-known fact that exercise, especially the aerobic kind, positively affects heart health. Heart disease is a significant killer, as plaque in the arteries begins to block the natural flow of blood. More than 600,000 in the U.S. die of heart disease, yet it is preventable. The primary causes are smoking, obesity, a poor diet, and inactivity. A yoga lifestyle usually eliminates all four of these factors to ensure better cardio health.

Many people avoid the word "exercise," imagining pumping madly in an aerobics class or jogging endlessly around a track.

These exercises are undoubtedly beneficial, but they aren't the only ones that can help us maintain a healthy heart and longer life.

With its gentle yet challenging poses, Yoga can bring about the benefits of aerobic exercise in an easier way.

There have been numerous studies comparing Yoga to no exercise and comparing Yoga to regular aerobic exercises.

Yoga practitioners showed straightforward and tremendous improvements in heart health compared to people who engaged in no physical exercise or exertion. They lost weight and achieved significantly lower blood pressure. Their cholesterol level also improved.

These results were expected. The surprise came when people practicing Yoga were compared to people who engaged in regular aerobics. There were no significant differences between the two groups in weight loss, cholesterol level, or blood pressure. The yoga group achieved the same level of benefits as the aerobics group.

A group of independent researchers, the Cochrane Collaboration, confirmed the results but indicated that the duration per week spent on practicing Yoga affects the long-term. People who attend a weekly yoga class will enjoy fewer benefits than those who practice Yoga several times a week or daily.

Many Americans suffer from atrial fibrillation, an irregular heart rhythm caused by high blood pressure, stress, and excess weight. Like common heart disease, atrial fibrillation, too, can be prevented.

A study at the University of Kansas used 52 patients suffering from atrial fibrillation and had them engage in two weekly yoga sessions for several months. The study results found that the participants enjoyed an improved heart rhythm and lessening anxiety and blood pressure.

Recent evidence suggests that Yoga, when practiced regularly, produces the same heart benefits as traditional aerobic exercises.

Transcendental meditation is a type of yoga meditation we will discuss in a further chapter. A study by the American Heart Association found that transcendental meditation can lower the risk of cardio death in almost half of the patients with heart problems.

Another study at the Medical College of Wisconsin assigned half of a group of patients with high blood pressure to a transcendental meditation group and had the other half taking blood pressure medication. The meditation group practiced 20 minutes a day for up to five years.

The study showed that almost half of the meditation group reduced heart problems compared to medication.

Further studies are being conducted. But there is clear evidence that Yoga has a significant positive impact on heart health.

Yoga and Weight Management

While there are quicker ways to lose weight, Yoga can help you shed a few pounds.

Yoga doesn't burn the same number of calories as aerobic exercise. You'll burn around 150 calories doing an hour of Yoga, which you'll burn over 300 doing an hour of walking.

But there's more to weight loss than just burning calories, though Yoga does provide a healthy workout. There is another, subtler, influence, however. Yoga increases awareness of our bodies and the food we use to fuel them. If your diet consists of burgers and chips, the enhanced mind/body connection will reinforce the toxicity of certain foods and make you reach for healthier, more life-affirming choices. Toxic food simply becomes less appealing. This means that most people will run for a salad instead of a burger.

If you want to lose weight on your yoga regime, opt for the more strenuous types of Yoga, such as Kundalini Yoga and Yin Yoga.

Chapter 6:

Different Types of Yoga

There are so many different types of yoga disciplines, and it can be not very clear to pick one. Don't let the variety stop you from diving into the yoga pool. Certain yoga types are geared toward beginners, and these are your best option when learning about the movements.

Also, keep in mind that the teacher can make or break the experience. If you don't feel comfortable in a particular class, it may be the instructor rather than the Yoga. Explore until you find your perfect yoga fit.

To begin Yoga at home, you will need a mat, yoga blocks, or towel for support, when needed, and a strap to use as a prop in certain bending poses.

Hatha Yoga

Hatha yoga is the most general type of Yoga and perhaps the most difficult to define. Depending on the teacher, classes can be slow and easy, but some may be more strenuous. To be sure a particular Hatha class is suitable for you, visit a level as a guest before signing up.

Hatha yoga consists of gentle movements without a continuing flow between each pose. This makes it easy for beginners to learn the basics. It is incredibly adaptable to individual needs and physical conditions and a great way to increase strength and flexibility while reducing the risk of injury.

It is the best place to start and learn the basic poses before moving on to more arduous movements and positions. The focus is on holding a pose and strengthening balance. Hatha yoga is slow-moving, so it isn't the best option if your goal is to move fast and sweat. The benefit of Hatha Yoga is a decrease in stress, and blood pressure as the body learns to relax.

Vinyasa Yoga

Vinyasa yoga has a quicker pace than Hatha, and poses can rapidly flow into each other, rather like dance steps. Each movement is linked to an inhale and exhale, thus linking movement with breathing. The mind remains focused and in the present.

There are no strict sequences to poses, and teachers can "mix and match" to vary the routine; therefore, if a particular Vinyasa class doesn't appeal to you, another might. Vinyasa yoga is less gentle than Hatha and pushes the boundaries of flexibility and strength. It provides a beautiful cardio workout, as your body is continuously moving, except when doing the restful Downward Dog. It is sure to work up a sweat. Relaxing music is frequently played in the background.

Like Hatha, Vinyasa is an excellent starting point for beginner-level yoga students.

Iyengar Yoga

Iyengar yoga is an extension of Hatha Yoga specifically focused on bodily alignment and can be tremendously healing. It increases flexibility through slow stretching moves that are held for some time. These still moments have meditative qualities. It tones the muscles and calms the mind. Better alignment can strengthen muscles, help with pain, and improve posture.

Iyengar yoga involves the entire body and improves circulation and digestion. With a better, healthier body, better lifestyle choices usually follow.

This form of Yoga may use chairs, belts, or other props to improve bodily alignment. It is perfectly appropriate for beginners.

Ashtanga Yoga

Ashtanga Yoga is more structured than some of the other asanas. There are six movements, six in all, and each series must be mastered before moving on to the next.

Ashtanga Yoga is not for beginners. It challenges strength, endurance, and flexibility; therefore, it is best to begin Ashtanga Yoga after familiarity with other yoga disciplines.

Ashtanga works the entire body so that results will come quickly. It does require commitment, and most practitioners of Ashtanga do the exercises every day. Each series can take years to master. Patient people will love Ashtanga because it requires repetition of the same poses. There is no variation until you reach the next level.

Bikram Yoga

There are 26 poses to be completed in a structured sequence for each Bikram session, which lasts for 1 hour and a half.

The twist to Bikram is that it is practiced in 105 degrees heat. You will sweat and will need to remain hydrated. The heat, of course, adds challenge. It also adds benefits, such as ridding the body of toxins.

Hot Yoga

As the name implies, Hot Yoga is also performed in a room filled with high temperatures. It differs from Bikram in that Hot Yoga is unstructured, without the 26 specific poses. This makes it suitable for beginners, but do consider the added challenge presented by the heat.

Kundalini Yoga

Kundalini uses meditation to energize the body. Its effects on the mind are potent as it increases awareness and strengthens your inner self to allow for a more authentic *you*. This harks back to Yoga's beginnings in its quest for spiritual elevation. Kundalini Yoga blends movements with breathing and chants.

Yin Yoga

Yin Yoga combines the physical with the mental and is specifically designed to provide energy and calm a busy mind.

The benefits of regular practice are a sense of calm, reduction in stress, improved circulation and flexibility, and greater joint mobility. The principle behind Yin Yoga is the yin and yang concept of Taoism, which seeks to balance all opposites in nature.

The exercises are done on the floor and involved holding poses for an extended time. This affects the lower body parts, specifically the hips, thighs, and spine.

Postures may be held for five minutes or more.

In a world that assaults us with stimuli continuously, the mind quickly becomes overloaded and overwhelmed. This is considered "normal" to such an extent people pride themselves on being Type A personalities. They are filled with a sense of urgency to always be on the move. The body is unable to relax, and the mind cannot become quiet.

Yin Yoga brings balance back to mind and body. The long poses stretch the tissues and strengthen the body while allowing awareness into the mind. Much energy is expended in suppressing unwanted thoughts and emotions. Yin Yoga releases that energy.

Restorative Yoga

Restorative Yoga restores your mind and body. It is easy, slow-moving, with poses held longer to provide a state of utter relaxation. Props such as blocks may be used to help you hold on to your posture.

Restorative Yoga helps you slow down when everything around you becomes hectic. Think of it as an isle of tranquility in a crazy world.

Chapter 7:

Attaining Better Immunity with Yoga Poses

A healthy immune system is the body's first defense against inflammation and diseases, from cancer to the flu. To function properly, your immune system needs to be in balance. That means that cells, organs, and tissues work together as an army, ready to defend the body against invaders, such as germs and other impurities. The immune system produces antibodies to help heal infections and rid the body of toxins.

Ever wonder why some people catch every bug making the rounds while others appear to be immune? Times of stress can render our immune system especially vulnerable. That is why the healthier our immune system, the quicker we can overcome the effects of bacteria, germs, and toxins. Healthy cells immediately come to our defense and attack those invaders. These helpful soldiers are the white blood cells.

Yoga is a natural relaxant and stress reliever and an excellent way to keep our immune system at an optimal level. It provides that necessary boost during times of stress.

Scientists have been studying the connection between Yoga and the immune system. A study in the Journal of Behavioral Medicine indicates that Yoga can help lessen inflammation. In 15 separate trials, researchers tested whether the practice of Yoga would affect inflammation. Most of the studies were done using easy Hatha poses. These studies showed a pattern that Yoga did decrease inflammation and had a positive effect on the body.

The best yoga programs were those that lasted up to 12 weeks of hourly sessions. The consistent practice was the key to success.

Besides inflammation, specific asanas can help release the irritation of the common cold, such as the Tortoise Pose.

Tortoise Pose

Sit with your buttocks and legs pressed into the floor. Stretch your legs open. Inhale, and lower your torso close to the floor as you exhale. Feel the stretch in your spine and inner thighs. Keep the pose for ten breaths.

Place your hands beneath your knees and take hold of each leg.

Depending on how flexible you are, you can lean forward as far toward the floor as possible, but don't force it. Inhale to expand your chest and exhale as you fold your body downward.

For sinus congestion, the Downward Dog (see Poses) can help alleviate congestion. This downward-bending pose also helps with infections as it drains the lungs.

Camel Pose for Bronchitis

If you suffer from bronchial congestion, the Camel pose can open up the body to allow you to breathe easier.

The Camel Pose will also help with neck and back pain. The Camel Pose can be strenuous on your back, so check with your doctor before getting started.

Start by stretching your spine by doing the Cobra Pose. This is an excellent warm-up and will prevent too much strain on the range. The Camel Pose is a challenging pose to master immediately, so take your time and work your way up to the full backward extension.

Remember, no yoga pose is ever forced. Kneel on a mat with hands on your hips. Tuck in your chin and press your tailbone toward the floor. Arch your pelvis forward.

If needed, place your hands by your tailbone.

This is an easy, modified Camel Pose. Once you have mastered it, you can bring your arms back and grab your heels. Remain in the Camel Pose for 60 seconds, or until you begin to feel uncomfortable.

Whatever type of Yoga you are currently practicing will help strengthen your immune system. The above forward and backward bends are simply extra helpful in giving your design a needed hand.

Yoga Poses

There are approximately 84 asanas, and this chapter will introduce you to a few of the basic ones. A few dos and don't before you start your journey:

- Do wear comfortable clothes.

- Don't practice asanas on a full stomach.

- Don't force any poses to the point of pain. Yoga is painless and should feel comfortable. Your flexibility and strength will improve with practice.

Mountain Pose

This is your starting point for all standing poses. It may look easy as if you're simply standing there, but it is intended to make you feel grounded.

Stand straight with your feet naturally apart. Press all ten toes into the ground. Raise your kneecaps and inner thighs for an upward lift. Tuck in your stomach and raise your chest. Keep your shoulders down.

Hold the palm of your hands toward your body. Inhale and feel your chest rise further. Hold the pose for 5 seconds.

Cat Pose

This is one of Yoga's most famous poses. Get down on your hands and knees, making sure your knees are aligned with your shoulders. Keep your head neutral.

Exhale and raise your spine and your head down. Inhale and lower your range and raise your head to the ceiling. Do this several times.

Downward Dog

Another favorite animal pose among yoga enthusiasts, this pose provides a beautiful stretch.

Go down on your hands and knees and keep your hands flat on the floor.

Inhale and raise your knees. Your heels will lift. Lift your tailbone toward the ceiling.

During the exhale, lower your heels to the floor and straighten the knees until your legs are straight. Keep your arms firm as you straighten them.

Warrior I Pose

Exhale and spread your feet about 4 feet apart. Lift your arms until they are perpendicular to the floor.

Shift the left foot 60 degrees to the right and the right foot 90 degrees to the right. The heels should be aligned.

Exhale and bend the right knee over the right ankle. With practice, your right thigh will be parallel to the floor.

Raise the ribcage and press down on your left foot. You should feel the stretch up the back of your left leg to your belly. Bring the palms of your hands together.

Remain in this pose for 30 seconds. Inhale, push the back heel into the floor and reach up and straighten the right knee.

Take a deep breath and reverse the legs and repeat the exercise.

Extended Puppy Pose

This pose stretches the spine as it soothes the mind. Get on your hands and knees.

Move your hands forward and curl toes under.

Exhale and bring your buttocks back to your heels. Keep your arms stretch forward while keeping your elbows off the ground.

With your buttocks above your heels, lower your forehead to the floor. Feel your spine stretch. Breathe into your spine and hold the pose for 30 seconds.

Triangle

The Triangle stretches and tones the entire body. Stand with your feet far apart. Lift both arms to shoulder height.

Turn the right foot out by 90 degrees and the other foot in by 45 degrees. Lower your right hand to your knee, or if you are able, touch your ankle. Raise your other hand to the ceiling.

Hold the pose for eight breaths, then repeat the exercise with the other side.

Cobra

Lay on the floor with your face down. Your legs are stretched behind without touching. Rest your hand's palms down beneath your shoulder while your fingers are pointing forward.

Inhale as you pull your chest and head upward as your arms straighten and your hands keep pressing into the floor. As you raise your chest, hold your shoulders back.

Don't force any lift that doesn't come naturally.

Hold the Cobra Pose for up to 30 seconds.

Tree Pose

The Tree Pose helps achieve and maintain balance while standing on one foot. This is an excellent asana for beginners.

Start by standing with your feet together. Raise your right foot as high as you can to the upper left thigh. Lift your hands and press the palms together. Keep looking ahead while maintaining your balance.

Plank Pose

Move to the Plank Pose from the Downward Dog. Inhale and lift your torso forward until your elbows are on the floor.

Press your lower arms into the floor and gaze at the bottom.

Hold the Plank Pose for 30 seconds and work up to 1 minute. This pose is designed to build strength. Keep breathing and make sure your shoulders are relaxed.

Chapter 8:

How to Get Started Doing Yoga?

As you start your yoga journey, it is necessary to keep in mind how important your mental attitude is for success. Bodily agility and flexibility will come with practice. But to begin practicing, you need the correct mindset.

For a beginner, it can be very confusing. Just picking out the right yoga outfit can be a headache! Then, how do you decide which yoga practice is the best one for you?

So, start by relaxing and consider following your roadmap to successful yoga practice.

Rid Yourself of Expectations

If you have viewed pictures of yoga poses and have decided that you could never achieve that type of agility, keep in mind that it undoubtedly took years, perhaps decades, for the model to get to that level. He or she was specifically chosen for his or her expertise.

Yoga is not about achieving the perfect pose. It's all about improved breathing and alignment. One step at a time, and the rest will follow. If you can't touch your toes, touch your knees instead. Toss any expectations you may have and start with an open mind. Yoga is non-judgmental; it is not a competition. Although with practice, you *will* naturally improve.

Age and body shape are mental limitations and do not affect your ability to begin a yoga practice. If you are physically unable to do a particular pose, there are dozen other poses you can master.

Find the Right Teacher

As you've probably figured out in high school and college, the right teacher can make a huge difference in any class. If you don't feel motivated and inspired by your yoga class, perhaps the teacher is wrong for you. This doesn't mean the teacher is terrible in any way, but he or she is not helping you meet your goals.

Consider whether the teacher is teaching things that you need to learn. Regardless of how good the teacher is, if he or she isn't helping you meet your needs, look for another one. Your best friend may rave about her Hot Yoga class, but you need to keep looking for another level if this isn't for you. Perhaps you want something less physical and more spiritual. There are plenty of yoga teachers out there, and one will be just right for you.

Are you moving toward your goal? A good teacher will guide you step by step along the journey. If you feel at a standstill, perhaps the teacher is not for you.

Can you ask questions? A good yoga teacher is available before and after class for his or her students and will listen and address individual concerns. If your teacher is not approachable, find one who is.

Don't hesitate to ask your teacher about his or her training or philosophy. The best type of teacher views Yoga as a continuous work-in-progress and is still studying with his or her teacher.

It's the Yoga, Not the Outfit

Do you know one of the primary reasons people don't go or stop going to the gym? They feel self-conscious among a group of perfect bodies.

Yoga has become so trendy; people are fretting which designer outfit is best and what color they should buy.

Do you need $125 Dior pants to attain enlightenment? Wear whatever feels comfortable. And don't compare yourself to anyone else. Yoga is a personal journey. As has been stated in this book before, it is not a competition.

All you need for Yoga is a simple pair of leggings, shorts, tank top, or T-shirt. Seriously, you're not trying to make a fashion statement. The only thing you need to keep in mind is comfort. Unique outfits are available for Hot Yoga.

You'll want a yoga mat that lasts, so do choose a quality mat. It will be an excellent investment.

Yoga Classes

Some yoga classes can cost up to $20.00. This can add up, but it shouldn't be a deterrent to getting started. There are ways to practice Yoga on a budget.

The local YMCA, gyms, and some community centers frequently offer yoga classes at low rates. During warm weather, yoga groups may meet at local parks.

When signing up for classes, buy in bulk. Signing up for 20 courses at a time instead of for individual courses may get you a discounted rate.

Some yoga studios rent mats and water bottles. They may only charge a dollar or so, but the extra expense can add up. Bring your mat and bottled water from home.

Some yoga studios offer "Karma Yoga" classes. These classes are free in exchange for doing some work at the studio, such as operating the front desk and cleaning up after a class. If cost is a concern, don't hesitate to ask about this option. Some studios will be happy to trade a course for a bit of service rendered.

The Best Time to Practice Yoga

A handy excuse not to get started with yoga practice is time. The fact is, we are all busy. We all have the same 24-hour day. If we intend to accomplish something, we need to *make* time.

Traditional Yoga involves sunrise or sunset. But using any time for Yoga is better than no yoga at all, although practicing Yoga on a full stomach is not a good idea. Get up an hour earlier than usual and do your asanas before you do anything else. It energizes and activates your body and mind in the best possible way. The physical poses get your body going, while breathing clears the mind.

Yoga Intentions

Some yoga teachers ask you to set your intentions at the start of the program. What exactly does that mean?

Setting an intention is not needed for you to enjoy the benefits of your yoga sessions. But it can take them to a higher level.

Setting your yoga intention brings Yoga into your daily life. Yoga doesn't stop when the asanas are done. They are supposed to be the beginning of your spiritual journey, not the end. Yoga was initially developed as a spiritual quest. The rest followed.

Intentions clarify your purpose in practicing Yoga. It focuses on a personal quality that you wish to improve or enhance.

Perhaps you hope for more incredible patience, awareness, or compassion toward others. Maybe you wish to let go of past hurts. Make that objective in your mind.

Your intentions are the bridge between your poses and the rest of your life. Yoga is not like walking out of the gym and forgetting about it until the next class. Mental practice should become a part of your daily life. You will set your mind to make it real by keeping your intentions in focus. That is genuine spiritual elevation.

Before You Begin, Talk to Your Doctor

Anyone can indeed practice Yoga. However, it would help if you discussed any possible limitations with your doctor before getting started. This won't prevent you from doing Yoga, but it might simply limit a few movements to avoid injury. Your doctor might also have some ideas about which type of Yoga is best for you. Having a doctor who is knowledgeable and supportive of Yoga is a tremendous asset.

Slow and Easy Does It

If Yoga is a new experience for you, it is natural to be excited and jump right in. But the goal of Yoga is not who can do the most poses in the least amount of time. Yoga is a slow and deliberate process. Each session should be devoted to making poses easier. Work at your level of comfort. It cannot be stressed enough that Yoga is non-competitive.

If certain poses are more complex than others, practice them more until they become more manageable. There is no time limit for mastering yoga poses. When poses become easier, go a bit beyond your comfort zone to reach the next level, but never to the point of physical discomfort.

Begin at Your Starting Point

Joining a new yoga class, where everyone else seems to know what they are doing, can be intimidating. But, that is the case when you begin any new endeavor.

Regardless of anyone else, you are your starting point. It is entirely irrelevant that everyone else can balance on one leg for 60 seconds while you keep tipping over. Instead of fretting, enjoy the progress as you keep improving. Savor who you are every step along the way. Self-acceptance is the essence of enlightenment.

The spiritual side of Yoga encourages compassion. Start with yourself.

Chapter 9:

Preventing Injuries

Practicing Yoga is as safe as walking. That being said, injuries are still possible, and you should take care to avoid them.

Start by following a few basic rules. Don't practice Yoga on a full stomach and avoid alcohol. Remain hydrated at all times.

Every yoga class should begin with warm-up exercises. If yours does not, look into another category. As we've discussed, the right teacher makes a tremendous difference and can reduce your chances of injury. Certified teachers undergo up to 500 hours of training to qualify for certification. Make sure you are dealing with a qualified teacher.

Don't try to do poses for which you aren't ready. This can cause severe muscle strain. Attempting poses for which you are unprepared is one of the leading causes of yoga injuries. Learn your body's limitations and respect them. You decide how far to stretch, not your teacher.

You may be feeling more agile on specific days than on others. If you are having a bad day, accept it and don't attempt challenging poses that may have been possible at other times. Listen to your body.

Certain areas of the body, such as the neck, lower back, knees, and hamstrings, are particularly vulnerable to injuries. Take care with any poses involving those body parts.

It is easy to become lightheaded when changing poses, so be sure to remain hydrated at all times.

Most yoga poses can be modified by using blocks or towels. Don't hesitate to use these modifications until your body can create the poses more effortlessly.

Don't begin Yoga by jumping into challenging poses, such as a headstand. This can cause severe neck injury. Work your way up to the more challenging poses.

Chapter 10:

Yoga and Meditation

Yoga is the bridge between meditation and spirituality. The original Buddhists used Yoga as a means to prepare for meditation. Meditation, like Yoga itself, is secular. Anyone can practice it. The purpose is to quiet, loud mental chatter and calm the mind.

Benefits of Meditation

1. Meditation allows you to become more aware of your inner and outer life. You start to notice emotions and thoughts that you may have previously denied.

2. It provides insight to improve your relationships.

3. Being aware helps you act at the moment instead of acting out of habit. Negative emotions can have you work in harmful ways, even when you are unaware of the reason for your behavior. When you become aware of these feelings, you can positively deal with them.

4. Meditation allows you to be less critical of yourself and others.

5. Meditation keeps you from acting on random emotions and lets you analyze facts before taking action.

6. Meditation reduces stress and anxiety.

7. Meditation helps you adapt to changing circumstances.

How Does Meditation Work?

Much research has been done on meditation for the past decades. Physically, meditation lowers our blood pressure and calms our nervous system. When we meditate, our heart rate and breathing slow down.

Through greater awareness, meditation allows us to change the way we think about past experiences. If you were continuously put down as a child, you began to accept it as usual. As an adult, those same feelings are still deep within you. You expect to be put down, even if there is no reason for such expectation. Regular meditation can change that negativity to allow you to accept more positive thoughts and emotions.

Studies have revealed that meditation can change our brain structure. People who meditate have enhanced areas dedicated to awareness and focus. Research at Harvard University has shown that while age can diminish certain brain regions, regular meditators retain the brain capacity of someone decades younger. For anyone seeking a higher level of existence, meditation has much to offer.

Another Harvard study showed that with regular meditation, areas of the brain that deal with fear and anxiety were reduced, while empathy and compassion areas became enlarged. Changing how our brain reacts is the ultimate in taking control of our lives.

How to Start Meditating

Like Yoga, meditation requires commitment. It is an ongoing process. The more we meditate, the better we get, and there are no limits to how well we can meditate. Ancient and current Buddhists spend a lifetime on meditation and self-empowerment.

Meditation requires a quiet place. Most people close their eyes and focus on their breathing, noticing every inhale and exhale. While other thoughts may intrude, they are simply acknowledged and set aside in a non-judgmental way. Start with just a few minutes – it is surprisingly difficult to sit quietly for any length of time because we are used to being constantly active. Work your way up to half an hour or forty-five minutes.

Try to meditate at the same time every day so that it becomes a daily habit. Find a comfortable place where you won't be disturbed. Meditating after getting up in the morning can get your day started on a positive note; however, meditating before going to bed can help you sleep better. Of course, there is no reason you can't meditate during both times of the day.

Finding Time to Meditate

Claiming not to have enough time is simply an excuse not to get started. You don't own time; you make it by getting up half an hour earlier in the morning. If you have your own office, close the door during lunchtime and use the hour, or part of it, for meditating. Do you spend a lot of time on social media? Limit your time, and you've bought yourself at least an hour or two every day.

Mindful Meditation

One of the most valuable types of meditation is mindful meditation. It brings greater awareness to our thought and emotions. Many people are chained to negative reviews, frequently about occurrences from years past. No matter how much time has passed, these emotions can still control our actions.

Mindful meditation allows us to acknowledge those negative feelings, then put them aside so that they no longer have the power to control us.

Mindful meditation is based on one critical hypothesis that cannot be overstated: **You Are Not Your Thoughts.**

Some people feel controlled by their negative emotions. Mindful meditation puts you in control. Like Yoga, meditation can change areas of the brain, increasing our ability for enjoyment and decreasing the sizes responsible for depression and anxiety.

Instead of having our minds jumbled with thoughts and feelings, mindfulness keeps us in the present to deal with what is happening *now.* This is a skill that can be learned.

How to Meditate Mindfully

Mindful meditation couldn't make it easier. If you can breathe, you can meditate. Simply follow a few simple steps and enjoy the relaxing benefits.

Find a quiet place, preferably with natural light. Ensure that you will not be disturbed. If you can find a peaceful place outdoors, it would be ideal.

A good amount of time to set aside for meditation is half an hour, but you can start with just five minutes and increase your time gradually. Like Yoga, it should be easy and not painful or uncomfortable.

Wear comfortable clothing. You don't want anything tight disrupting your meditative flow.

It is helpful to have a timer set to keep you from glancing at your watch.

You can use a chair or sit on the floor using cushions. If on the floor, cross your legs in a comfortable lotus position, which is the traditional Buddhist meditating stance. If you are sitting on a chair, have your feet touch the floor or use blocks on which to rest your feet.

Your torso should be straight but not stiff. Rest your hands on your thighs. You should feel comfortably at rest.

Most people prefer meditating with their eyes closed as it removes distractions. But if you prefer, you can leave them open.

Next, just relax. Gradually begin to focus on your breathing as you inhale and exhale deeply. Notice how the air feels going in and going out. Feel the rise and fall of your chest.

It is natural for your focus to wander as other thoughts enter your mind. There is no reason to get upset and pretend these thoughts aren't there. Acknowledge them and then return your focus to your breathing.

If your mind wanders a great deal, simply observe what is happening in a non-critical way. Please don't force them away; merely pay attention to what is happening.

One way to increase your focus is by counting. Inhale, count 1, exhale, count 2 ... up to twenty. Then trust in reverse.

Remain still for a few minutes after you have finished meditating. Notice how you feel, your thoughts, and your emotions. Become an observer, not a critic.

Meditation is as easy as this, yet it can bring about powerful changes. When practiced with Yoga, you will notice your mind and body working in natural harmony.

Conclusion

People have been practicing Yoga for thousands of years, and it is still attracting new advocates, especially those in the medical profession. There is no doubt that it has a lot to offer as we attempt to reach a higher level of existence.

1. Yoga is not a religious practice. Nevertheless, it does put us in touch with our spiritual essence. The original Buddhist yogis practiced Yoga to increase enlightenment and enhance their understanding of the world around them. Yoga was preparation for meditation. The origin of Yoga was far more spiritual than it is today, but it still enhances our spiritual self.

2. Yoga improves our immune system, heart rate, cardio health, circulation, and breathing. It reduces stress, anxiety and enhances flexibility and muscle tone. The benefits of Yoga can reduce the effects of aging both physically and mentally.

3. There are many different types of Yoga, some easy and gentle, while others are highly demanding. They all provide benefits, but we should choose the Yoga that is best for us.

4. Nothing about Yoga should be painful or forced. If you feel pain or discomfort

during yoga practice, talk to your teacher. You are either doing the exercise incorrectly, or you are in the wrong class. There are many classes from which to choose, so you never have to settle for one that makes you feel uncomfortable.

5. Yoga poses affect our entire body as they stretch our muscles to the limit. Unlike other exercises, which may focus only on specific body parts, yoga poses involve the body as a whole. That is why many consider Yoga superior to aerobics or weightlifting. Of course, aerobics and weights can be practiced in conjunction with Yoga for optical, physical benefits.

6. Yoga connects the mind with the body to create one functioning unit. We are well aware of how the reason can affect the body and our overall health. Negative thoughts can cause severe diseases and inflammations, such as arthritis. Yoga aims to clear the mind of negativity and bring optimal health back to the body. Never forget that the mind and body work together.

Use the following rules as the best way to approach your yoga sessions:

1. Everyone has his or her starting point, so don't worry about weight, age, or flexibility. Your poses will improve with practice, but they

should never compete with the rest of the class.

2. Finding the right teacher will make a big difference. A good teacher should answer questions and never force poses that are beyond the student's capability. If this is your experience, find another teacher.

3. Many people begin Yoga with certain expectations. However, everyone is different. You may never be able to do a headstand, while the rest of the class appears to do so with ease. That is perfectly okay. The only rule in Yoga is to work at your level of comfort. Nothing should ever be forced.

4. Start slowly. People practice Yoga for decades and are still striving for perfection. There is no perfect yoga pose. There is only you, your body, and your mind reaching ever-higher levels.

5. Before you begin a yoga class, check with your doctor. Yoga movements are safe, and injuries are rare, but you still want to ensure that there is nothing to prevent you from practicing Yoga safely.

6. Meditation is an essential part of Yoga. As we have discussed, ancient yogis used Yoga to prepare the body for their meditative practices. To get the complete physical, mental,

and spiritual benefits of Yoga, make meditation a part of your life.

7. Yoga can add much to your life and can help you become a better version of yourself.

CPSIA information can be obtained
at www.ICGtesting.com
Printed in the USA
BVHW041525160621
609641BV00013B/3013

9 781803 120393